The Economic Benefits of the Affordable Care Act

Remarks by Jason Furman[1]
Chairman, Council of Economic Advisers

Center for American Progress
April 2, 2015

Expanded prepared remarks

It is great to be back at the Center for American Progress (CAP) with my friend Neera Tanden. CAP has been a powerful advocate for progressive policies, so it is fitting that I am here to discuss the economic benefits of the Affordable Care Act, one of the most significant pieces of progressive legislation in decades—and one that gave me the great opportunity of working closely with Neera.

Paul Krugman recently argued that the direct benefits of the Affordable Care Act for the health and financial security of Americans are so large that just establishing that the Affordable Care Act did not do any economic harm would be sufficient to justify it. But I believe we can do even better and today I want to talk about the many ways that the Affordable Care Act has benefited—and will benefit—our economy by expanding health insurance coverage and reforming our health care delivery system in ways that reduce health costs and improve quality of care.

But before I get to this affirmative case, it is worth spending a moment reflecting on what the law has not done. During the debate over the law and the years that followed, we heard a stream of predictions that the law would cause economic catastrophe. To put it mildly, these doomsday prophecies have not come to pass.

One popular claim has been that the law would be a "job killer." To the contrary, starting with the month the Affordable Care Act became law, our businesses have created 12 million new jobs over 60 months of continuous job growth, the longest streak of private sector job growth on record. And over the last twelve months as the Affordable Care Act's main coverage provisions have begun to have their full effect, we have created 3.2 million private sector jobs, the strongest twelve-month period of private sector job growth since 1998. And, from 2013 to 2014, the unemployment rate declined by 1.2 percentage points, the largest annual decline since 1984.

---

[1] Matt Fiedler led the preparation of this speech with assistance from Gabe Scheffler.

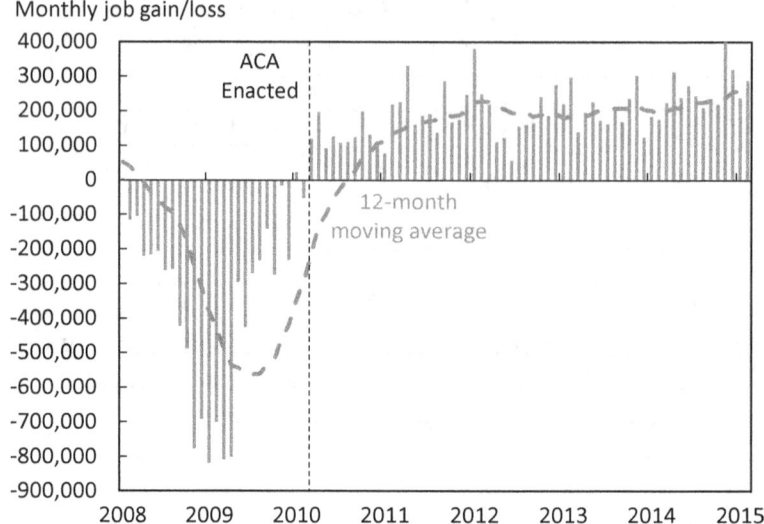

Figure 1
Private Sector Payroll Employment

Others said that the law would create a "part-time economy" and drive a major shift toward part-time work. This too has turned out to be false. Since the Affordable Care Act became law, 101 percent of overall increase in employment has been in full-time jobs. In other words, part-time employment has actually declined slightly, even as overall employment has grown steadily.

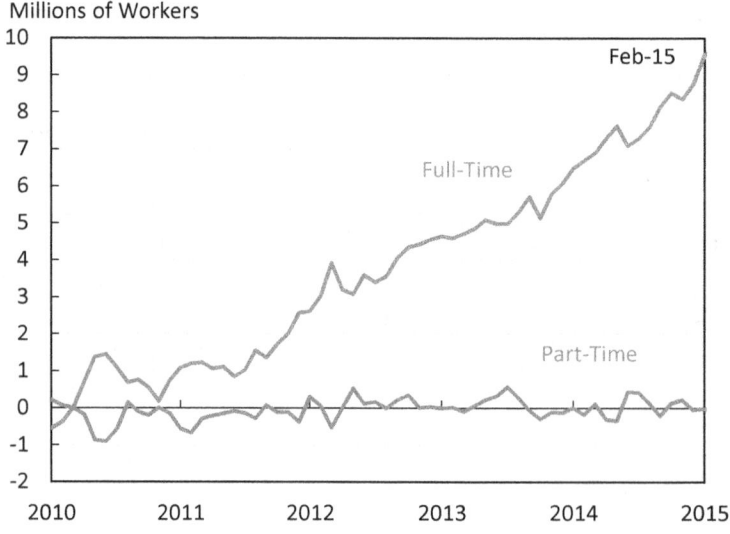

Figure 2
Net Change in Employment Since March 2010

Likewise, many claimed that the law that was a "budget buster" that would explode deficits. To the contrary, over the past several years, we have seen the Federal deficit fall by more than two-thirds as a share of the economy. And, more to the point, the Congressional Budget Office (CBO) has consistently predicted that the law will reduce deficits, particularly long-term deficits, generating savings of more than $1 trillion over two decades. If anything, the law's fiscal effects are looking better than originally anticipated. Since March 2010, CBO has reduced its estimate of the long-term cost of the law's coverage provisions by about one-third, as shown in Figure 3.

Figure 3

Net Cost of the ACA Coverage Provisions, 2015-2019

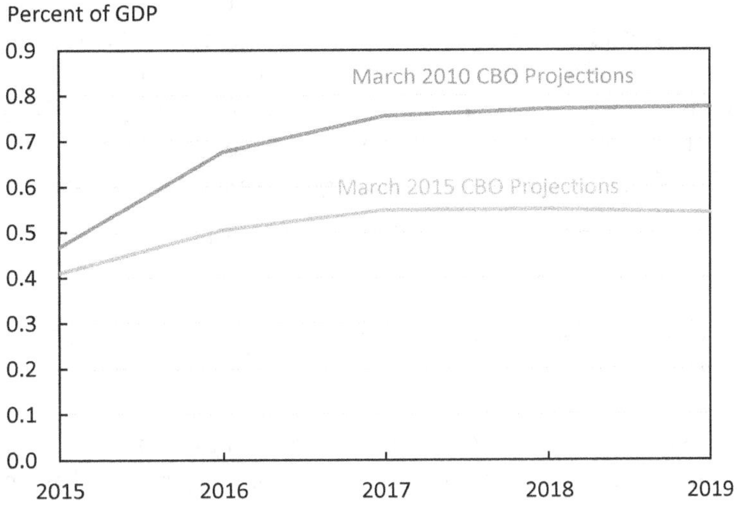

Percent of GDP

I could go on in this vein, but, as I noted above, my goal today is not to respond to the most overheated charges that have been leveled against the law in the past, but instead to discuss the real economic benefits the law is generating today and will generate in the future.

I will examine in turn each of the two main prongs of the law. First, I will examine the law's provisions *expanding insurance coverage* and how those provisions benefit our economy by creating a healthier, more productive workforce, reducing job lock to help people structure their careers in more economically efficient ways, and providing needed support in downturns in order to speed economic recoveries—including the current recovery.

Second, I will examine recent trends in health care costs and quality and their relationship to the law's measures to *reduce costs and improve quality*. Since the Affordable Care Act was passed, we have seen the slowest growth in health care prices over any period of that length in nearly 50 years. And thanks to slow growth in per-enrollee health care spending across both the public and private sectors, the three slowest years of growth in real per capita national health expenditures on record were 2011, 2012, and 2013. At the same time, metrics of health care quality have improved—including a 17 percent reduction in hospital-acquired conditions since 2010 that corresponds to 50,000 avoided deaths from 2010 through 2013 and a sharp reduction in hospital readmissions that translates into 150,000 avoided readmissions in 2012 and 2013. Although these reductions in health cost growth and improvements in quality have many causes, there is no doubt that the Affordable Care Act is playing a role.

Third, I will talk about the economic benefits of these changes, particularly the implications for the job market and the fiscal outlook if even a portion of that slow health cost growth can be sustained. Strikingly, the average family premium in employer-based coverage was about $1,800 lower in 2014 than if growth since 2010 had matched the 2000-10 average, and that difference

3

will widen further if even a portion of the health slowdown continues. Moreover, the deficit reduction associated with the Affordable Care Act and subsequent downward revisions in CBO's projections of health care spending have been sufficient to cut the 25-year fiscal gap by more than half.

I will conclude by briefly discussing the Administration's ongoing efforts to widely deploy new ways of paying medical providers that reward efficient, high-quality care, rather than a high volume of care, efforts that would be catalyzed by the bipartisan, bicameral reforms to Medicare's physician payment system that were included in the President's Budget and recently passed by the House and that will soon be taken up in the Senate. These efforts likely constitute our best tool for ensuring that the slow health care cost growth seen in recent years continues in the years ahead.

The Benefits of the Historic Expansion in Health Insurance Coverage for Labor Markets and the Macroeconomy

One central goal of the Affordable Care Act is to ensure that all Americans have access to high-quality, affordable health insurance. Despite many attempts to achieve this goal over the last several decades, the last time that the United States actually made major progress on this front was in the middle of the twentieth century. Modern health insurance first developed in the United States in the late 1920s, and the market remained relatively small until 1940.[2] Following the Second World War, private health insurance spread rapidly, bringing health insurance to about three-quarters of the U.S. population by the early 1960s. The creation of Medicare and Medicaid in 1965 and their subsequent expansion to people with disabilities in 1972 helped drive continued rapid progress in expanding coverage through the late 1960s and early 1970s.

Figure 4
Percent of Population Without Health Insurance, 1963-2015:Q1

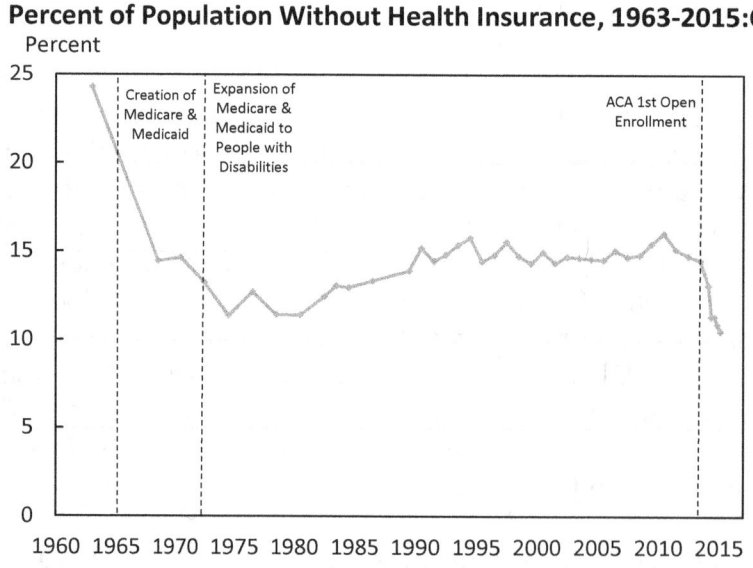

---

[2] Thomasson, Melissa. 2002. "From Sickness to Health: The Twentieth-Century Development of U.S. Health Insurance." *Explorations in Economic History*, vol. 39, pp. 233-253.

However, as shown in Figure 4, progress stalled starting in the mid-1970s. The uninsured rate rose during the 1980s and then moved sideways over the following two decades, with around 15 percent of Americans—47 million people in today's terms—lacking coverage at any given point in time. Many of these uninsured Americans were people with modest incomes who could not afford coverage. Others lacked access to coverage through the workplace and faced a broken individual insurance market in which getting affordable coverage was difficult or impossible, particularly for people with pre-existing medical conditions. State Medicaid expansions during the 1980s and 1990s and the creation of the Children's Health Insurance Program (CHIP) in 1997 helped to address these problems, particularly for children, but these positive steps were offset in the aggregate by ongoing erosion in private insurance.

The Affordable Care Act addressed the problem of widespread uninsurance in two main ways. First, it fixed the individual insurance market—using an approach patterned after earlier reforms in Massachusetts—by banning discrimination on the basis of pre-existing conditions, providing tax credits to low-, moderate-, and middle-income Americans to help them afford coverage, and requiring those who can afford to purchase coverage to do so. Second, the law provided financial support to States that elect to expand their Medicaid programs.

These provisions took effect at the beginning of 2014, and the results have been dramatic. Since the end of 2013, we have seen a precipitous decline in the uninsured rate, a decline unlike anything since the one following the creation of Medicare and Medicaid. Following this decline, the Nation's uninsured rate now stands at its lowest level ever. A recent analysis by the Department of Health and Human Services (HHS) indicated that, as of the early months of 2015, an estimated 16.4 million people have gained coverage, including both people who have gained coverage since the end of 2013 and young adults who gained coverage before 2014 due to the law's option to remain on a parent's plan until age 26.

More progress is likely over the coming months and years. The data in Figure 4 do not fully capture the gains made during 2015 open enrollment, so the uninsured rate is likely to decline somewhat further before the end of 2015. Likewise, independent analysts, including CBO, forecast further gains in future years as more people become aware of the option to obtain coverage through the Marketplaces or Medicaid and as more States elect to expand Medicaid.

Economic research demonstrates clearly that this expansion in coverage is generating major benefits for the newly insured by increasing access to needed care, improving health, and enhancing families' financial security. Since these direct economic benefits of expanded coverage are more widely understood, I will not dwell on them here, but I encourage those interested in learning more to CEA's report last year on the consequences of State decisions about whether to expand their Medicaid programs.[3] Rather, I will focus on three benefits of expanded coverage for the labor market that have received less attention.

---

[3] (CEA) Council of Economic Advisers. 2014. "Missed Opportunities: The Consequences of State Decisions Not to Expand Medicaid" (July).

First, by improving workers' access to care and their physical and—possibly particularly important—mental health, the Affordable Care Act is helping people live longer, healthier lives—which likely means that they will miss fewer days of work, be less likely to become disabled, spend more years in the workforce, and be more productive while on the job. Taken together, these benefits will make it easier for them to secure employment and boost earnings.

The notion that expanding health insurance coverage improves workers' labor market prospects is intuitive in light of the evidence that health insurance improves health status and the strong correlation between better health and employment documented in Figure 5. But clearly documenting a causal link has been difficult, likely in part because these effects appear only gradually over time. Indeed, the best evidence we have suggests that these effects are small in the short run. The Oregon Health Insurance Experiment, which arose from the State of Oregon's decision to address a funding shortage by allocating Medicaid coverage for low-income adults by lottery, found no evidence that access to health insurance drove near-term changes in earnings or the probability of being employed, either positive or negative.[4]

Figure 5

Percent of Working Age Adults Employed by Health Status

Percent of adults ages 25-64 who are employed

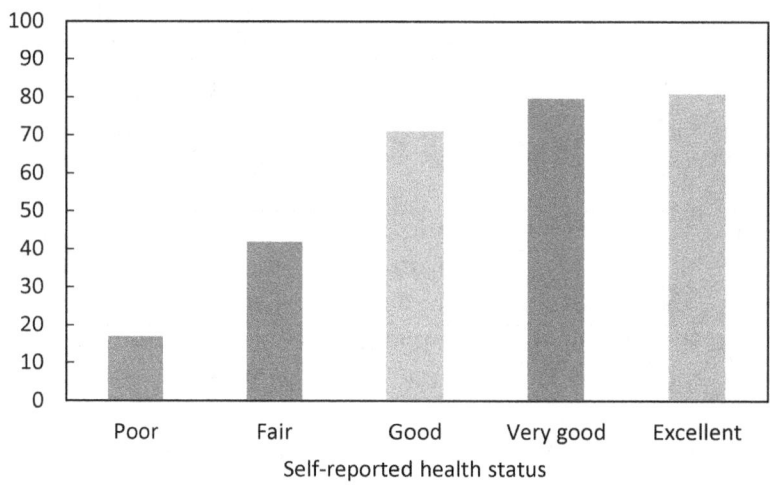

Self-reported health status

However, recent research suggests that the picture may look meaningfully different over the long run. These papers have examined the consequences of prior expansions of insurance coverage to children through Medicaid or the Children's Health Insurance Program (CHIP). Because many of these program expansions are now decades old, it is increasingly feasible to study how expanding access to health insurance through these programs has affected beneficiaries' outcomes as adults.

---

[4] Baicker, Katherine, Amy Finkelstein, Jae Song, and Sarah Taubman. 2013. "The Impact of Medicaid on Labor Force Activity and Program Participation: Evidence from the Oregon Health Insurance Experiment." NBER Working Paper 19547. October.

In particular, two recent studies have used variation in Medicaid/CHIP eligibility rules across states and over time to examine how Medicaid eligibility in childhood affects education and labor-market outcomes in adulthood. The first of these studies concludes that eligibility for Medicaid/CHIP coverage in childhood substantially increases children's probability of completing high school and college, presumably with attendant benefits for employment and earnings.[5] The second study finds similar evidence of improvements in educational attainment plus direct evidence of increased earnings in early adulthood, at least for women. It also finds evidence that both men and women pay more in income and payroll taxes in their young adult years, potentially offsetting a substantial fraction of the cost of providing Medicaid/CHIP coverage to children.[6]

The mechanism behind these long-run benefits is unclear, but a pair of complementary studies suggest that long-lasting improvements in health status are playing an important role. These studies use a feature of Federal Medicaid eligibility rules that caused children born in October 1983 or later to be more likely to qualify for Medicaid coverage during their pre-teen and early-teen years than children born before October 1983.[7] The authors find that, in the socioeconomic groups most affected by the discontinuity in coverage eligibility, children born on the October 1983 side of the eligibility threshold experience lower mortality in their late teen years and are substantially less likely to be hospitalized as adults. These findings imply that access to Medicaid coverage in childhood generated durable improvements in health, improvements that could improve their ability to participate in the labor market later in life.

To be sure, this evidence does not conclusively establish that health improvements generated by the Affordable Care Act's coverage expansion will improve long-run labor market outcomes for those gaining coverage. Notably, the studies I have just described examine coverage expansions affecting children, while the Affordable Care Act's coverage expansions primarily affect adults. Nevertheless, this research establishes that access to insurance coverage at a point in time can have important benefits for labor market outcomes much later in life, benefits that appear to be mediated at least in part through durable improvements in health. Together with the well-documented link between health insurance and health status and the strong intuitive case linking health status and labor market outcomes, it justifies a strong presumption that the Affordable Care Act's coverage expansions will have similar effects.

Reducing "Job Lock" and Improving Labor Market Flexibility

Second, by improving access to health insurance outside the workplace, the Affordable Care Act is reducing "job lock" and allowing workers to make employment choices based on what makes

---

[5] Cohodes, Sarah, Daniel Grossman, Samuel Kleiner, and Michael F. Lovenheim. 2014. "The Effect of Child Health Insurance Access on Schooling: Evidence from Public Health Insurance Expansions." NBER Working Paper 20178. May.

[6] Brown, David, Amanda Kowalski, and Ithai Lurie. 2015. "Medicaid as an Investment in Children: What is the Long-Term Impact on Tax Receipts?" NBER Working Paper 20835. January.

[7] Meyer, Bruce, and Laura Wherry. 2012. "Saving Teens: Using a Policy Discontinuity to Estimate the Effects of Medicaid Eligibility." NBER Working Paper 18309. August; Wherry, Laura, Sarah Miller, Robert Kaestner, and Bruce Meyer. 2015. "Childhood Medicaid Coverage and Later Life Health Care Utilization." NBER Working Paper 20929. February.

the most economic sense, rather than based on where they can get access to health insurance. Before the Affordable Care Act, most individuals' best option for obtaining health insurance coverage was through the workplace. Purchasing insurance coverage on the individual market was often unaffordable or even impossible, particularly for people with pre-existing conditions. This could trap workers in jobs that offered health insurance, rather than allowing them to make the employment choices that best matched their career and life plans.

By eliminating "job lock," the Affordable Care Act is improving economic efficiency in several concrete ways. It can, for example, allow people to structure their careers in ways that make sense for them, like by taking time off to raise a family or by retiring when they want to. It also allows people to take risks that further their careers and benefit the economy as a whole, like going back to school, leaving a job in order to start a business, or switching to a job that offers better opportunities for growth over the long term but does not offer health insurance.

The economic benefits of eliminating job lock may be particularly large for younger workers, both because they are particularly likely to want to take time out of the labor force to pursue schooling and because early-career job matches may have a large effect on long-term career trajectories. As shown in Figure 6, this group experienced large coverage gains even before 2014 due to the law's provision allowing young adults to stay on a parent's plan until age 26.

Figure 6

Young Adult Uninsured Rates, 1997:Q1-2013:Q4

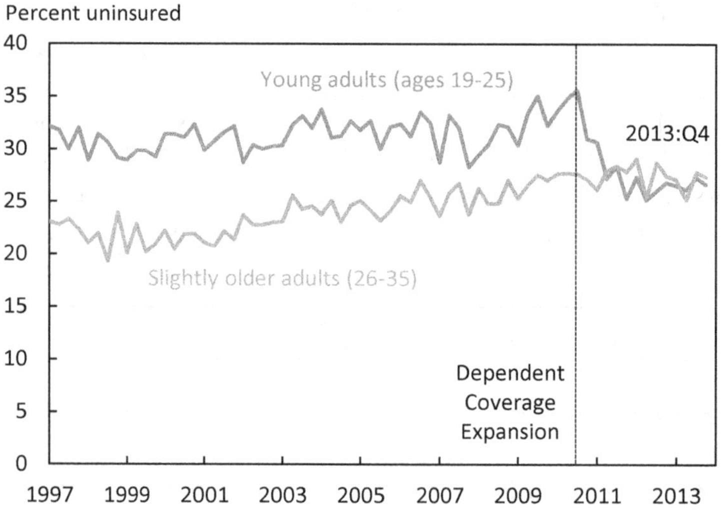

Intriguing evidence on the labor market benefits of reduced job lock for young adults comes from a recent study that examined pre-Affordable Care Act State laws that allowed some young adults to remain on a parent's plan at older ages.[8] These State laws were typically narrower than the Affordable Care Act provision since they did not apply if the young adult's parent received coverage through a self-insured employer. However, these laws have been in effect for a much longer period, making it possible to examine longer-term labor market consequences.

---

[8] Dillender, Marcus. 2014. "Do More Health Insurance Options Lead to Higher Wages? Evidence from States Extending Dependent Coverage." *Journal of Health Economics*, Vol. 36, pp. 84-97. July.

This study concluded that living in a State with a dependent coverage law during young adulthood increased educational attainment, at least for men, and boosted men's and women's wages later in adulthood by more than 1.5 percent on average. A 1.5 percent wage increase translates into about $650 per year for the typical full-time, year-round worker. Because the Affordable Care Act's coverage expansions benefit a broader swath of young adults (including young adults whose parents work at large employers or do not have coverage), its long-term labor market benefits could be even larger. While this study is not the last word on this topic, the results imply that the long-term economic benefits of reducing job lock for young adults may be quite substantial.

Better Macroeconomic Performance

Third, the law's coverage provisions are accelerating the labor market recovery by increasing families' demand for health care goods and services and by reducing their out-of-pocket medical costs, which frees up money to meet other pressing needs.[9] Since these provisions have taken effect at a time when the economy remains constrained by inadequate aggregate demand, they are likely boosting overall employment, consistent with predictions in early 2014 by then-CBO Director Doug Elmendorf that the law "would reduce unemployment over the next few years."[10]

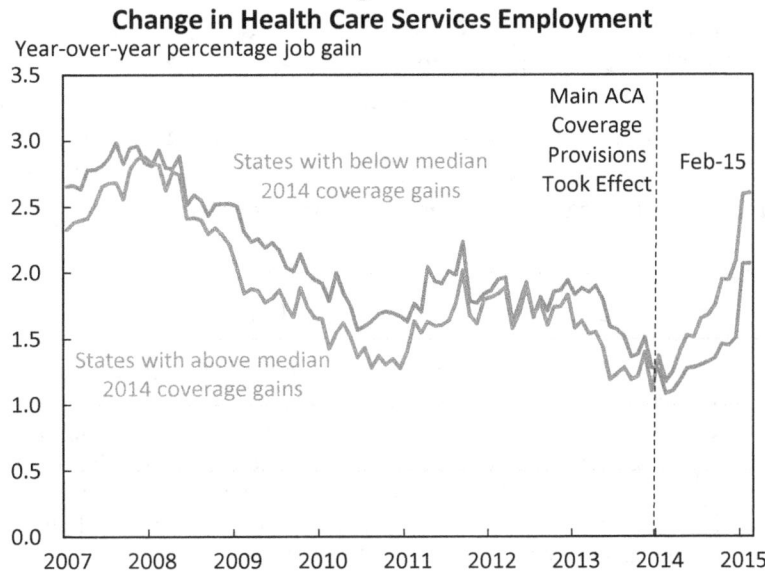

Figure 7
Change in Health Care Services Employment

---

[9] The Affordable Care Act is deficit-reducing overall, including in fiscal year 2014 and 2015, due largely to reductions in excessive payments to providers and insurers in Medicare, higher taxes on certain high-income individuals, and excise taxes on certain specific industries. On a dollar-for-dollar basis, the negative aggregate demand effects of these deficit-reducing provisions are likely considerably smaller than the effects of the positive effects of the law's coverage provisions since the entities affected by the deficit-reducing provisions are much less likely to use an additional dollar of cash on hand to increase consumption or investment today, implying that the law increases aggregate demand overall. Nevertheless, because the estimates presented below reflect the demand-side effects of the coverage provisions only, the effects of the law as a whole could be somewhat smaller.

[10] Elmendorf, Douglas. 2014. Testimony on the Congressional Budget Office's Budget and Economic Outlook before the House of Representatives Committee on the Budget. February.

We can see direct evidence of these effects by looking at data on health care services employment growth during 2014. As shown in Figure 7, health care employment growth picked up sharply in early 2014, and the pickup has been larger in the States experiencing larger gains in insurance coverage during 2014. The relationship between the extent of a State's coverage gains from 2013 to 2014 and its pickup in health care employment growth during 2014 implies that the decline in the uninsured rate from 2013 to 2014 boosted health care employment nationwide by about 0.9 percent as of February 2015, which translates to about 130,000 jobs.[11]

Economists generally do not view increasing health care employment as a goal of public policy since, when the economy is at full employment, each additional worker employed in the health care sector is a worker not available to produce other valued goods and services, and the goals of the Affordable Care Act were to expand coverage, slow the growth of health costs, and improve quality, not increase health care employment. But, in this case, the increase in health sector jobs is a positive development for two reasons. First, the Affordable Care Act's coverage expansion happened to take effect in an economy that remains short of full employment, so additional health sector employment will not come at the cost of reduced employment elsewhere in the economy in the short run. Second, additional health sector employment is appropriate if the benefits of the additional care provided is worth the cost, a condition that is almost certain to be satisfied in this case given the substantial benefits to the newly insured.

The increase in aggregate demand due to the law's coverage expansion is likely also creating jobs outside the health sector. By reducing families' out-of-pocket medical costs, the Affordable Care Act is directly increasing demand for non-health goods and services. Similarly, increases in health care employment will drive follow-on increases in demand in non-health sectors as the new health care workers spend their paychecks.[12] In sum, this suggests that the Affordable Care Act has contributed to the acceleration in overall job growth over the last year or so.

---

[11] The 95 percent confidence interval for this estimate stretches from a 0.3 percent increase to a 1.5 percent increase. This estimate was derived by regressing the 12-month change in the logarithm of health care employment on the percentage point change in the uninsured rate from 2013 to 2014 separately for each month from the beginning of 2013 through the present. The causal effect of changes in the uninsured rate on health care employment growth was then computed by comparing the estimated coefficients on the change in the uninsured rate during 2014 to the average coefficient during 2013. These estimates were then used to compute the cumulative difference through February 2015. For details on the data used, see the notes for Figure 7.

[12] Consistent with this theory, applying the same methodology used to estimate the effect of expanding coverage on health care employment suggests that the decline in the uninsured rate from 2013 to 2014 boosted total non-farm employment by about 220,000 jobs. However, in large part because non-farm employment is affected by many factors other than changes in the uninsured rate, this estimate is highly imprecise, and a 95 percent confidence interval includes both declines in employment and much larger gains. In addition, this methodology may be subject to various biases when used to study demand-side effects of expanded coverage on overall employment, biases that are not present when examining health care employment alone. For example, this approach could overstate the effect of expanding coverage on overall job growth to the extent that faster employment growth *causes* faster gains in insurance coverage by expanding access to workplace coverage, rather than the other way around. On the other hand, this comparison could understate the aggregate demand effects of expanded coverage since, unlike the health care employment gains which will typically occur locally, some portion of the non-health employment gains may occur in other States. In addition, some analysts expect the law to have effects on labor supply as workers reconfigure their working lives in response to the new coverage options made available under the law, effects that would also be captured in this estimate.

The boost that the Affordable Care Act is currently providing to overall employment will fade as the economy finishes healing from the Great Recession and aggregate demand returns to a normal level—a feature of all demand-side policies. But this is unlikely to be the last time that the Affordable Care Act provides a needed boost to aggregate demand. Recent discussions of macroeconomic policy have suggested that changes in the United States economy have increased the likelihood that monetary policy will be constrained by the zero lower bound in future recessions, raising the likelihood that fiscal policy will have to play an important role in combatting recessions in the future.[13]

That makes improvements in the United States' system of automatic stabilizers—programs that automatically expand during hard times and contract during good ones—particularly valuable. While the Affordable Care Act is not normally thought of as a countercyclical macroeconomic policy, it is just that. By safeguarding families' access to health care and cushioning household budgets in the face of the job and income losses that occur during a recession, the combination of the tax credits and the Medicaid expansion will help households smooth consumption and will expand aggregate demand when it would otherwise be impaired, reducing the severity of future recessions while better protecting families from their consequences.

The Role of the Affordable Care Act in Recent Slow Growth in Health Costs and Improvements in Health Care Quality

While one important goal of the Affordable Care Act is expanding access to health insurance coverage, another important goal is addressing long-standing shortcomings of our health care delivery system that have increased costs, while undermining health care quality. The health care sector is more than 17 percent of our economy, and the value of good health is difficult to overstate, so even modest inefficiencies—and almost everyone agrees the inefficiencies in our health care system have historically been much more than modest—substantially reduce Americans' standard of living and overall well-being. Here too, recent experience has been exceptionally encouraging.

Recent Trends in Health Costs

I will start with costs. In examining recent trends in health costs, it is useful to consider three different measures of health care costs: first, the unit prices of health care goods and services; second, average spending per enrollee in different types of health insurance coverage, which reflects both unit prices and per-enrollee utilization; and third, aggregate national health expenditures, which reflect both the number of people with health insurance coverage and average spending per covered person. Let me discuss each in turn.

Health care unit prices capture what is happening to the price of specific health care goods and services, like a tablet of aspirin or an appendectomy, and health care price indices aim to capture

---

[13] Summers, Lawrence. 2014. "U.S. Economic Prospects: Secular Stagnation, Hysteresis, and the Zero Lower Bound." *Business Economics*, vol. 49, no. 2, pp. 65-73. February; Teulings, Coen, and Richard Baldwin, eds. 2014. *Secular Stagnation: Facts, Causes and Cures*. London: Centre for Economic Policy Research.

the changing cost of purchasing a fixed basket of health care goods and services. Over the 59 months of data since the Affordable Care Act became law, these prices have risen at an average annual rate of 1.7 percent, the slowest pace for a period of this length in nearly 50 years, and the rate of health care price increases over the most recent 12 months has been an even slower 1.2 percent, as shown in Figure 8. The rate of increase in health care prices since the Affordable Care Act became law is only slightly faster than the 1.4 percent annual rate for all consumer goods and services over this period. This small a sustained differential between health care price inflation and overall inflation has been achieved on only two other brief occasions.

Figure 8

Health Care Price Inflation versus Overall Inflation

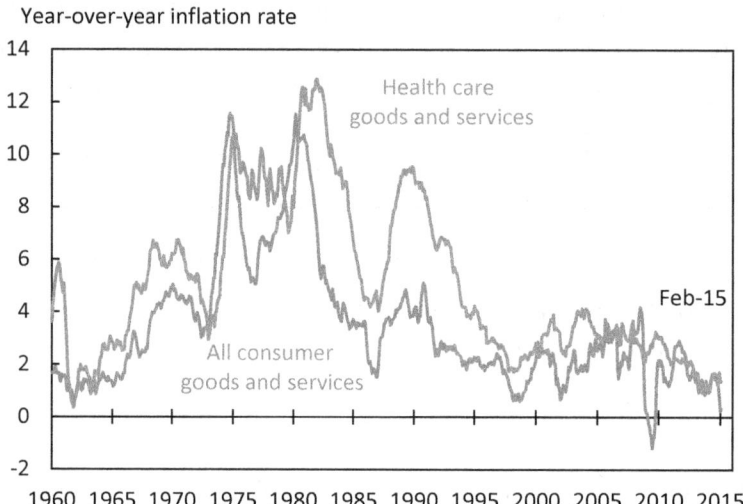

The average cost for an individual or a family depends on both the price of health care and the quantity of health care consumed—so it could, for example, go up because the cost of a CT scan rises or because each person with insurance uses more CT scans. Average health care spending per insured individual has also shown exceptionally slow growth in recent years, due both to the slow growth in health care prices described above and slow growth in the number of services used per insured individual. Slow growth in per-enrollee spending has been seen in both the public and private sectors, as depicted in Figure 9 using spending data that extend through 2013. While the comprehensive data underlying Figure 9 are not yet available for 2014, data on Medicare spending and employer health benefits costs, depicted in Figure 10, indicate that slow growth in per-enrollee costs has continued during 2014, despite some upward cost pressure from a wave of expensive new prescription medications entering the market.[14]

---

[14] Near-real-time data on per-enrollee spending in Medicaid are not available, and, in any case, would be distorted by the ongoing coverage expansion, which is adding millions of largely healthy adults to the program.

Figure 9

Growth in Real Per Enrollee Spending by Payer

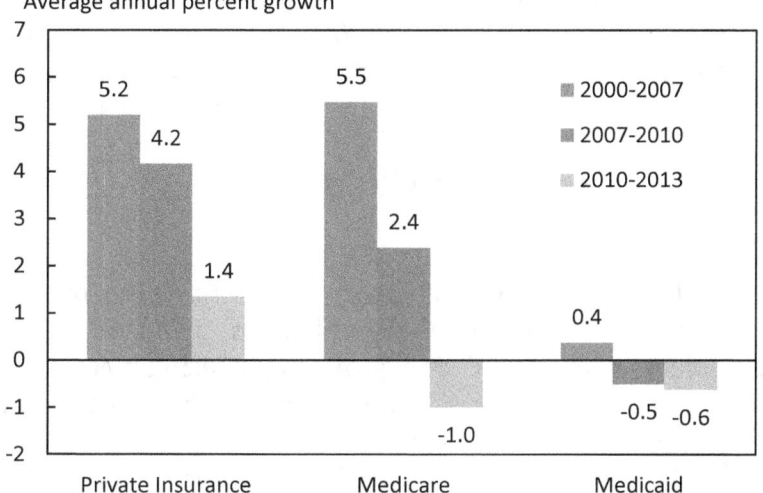

Average annual percent growth

- 2000-2007
- 2007-2010
- 2010-2013

Private Insurance: 5.2, 4.2, 1.4
Medicare: 5.5, 2.4, -1.0
Medicaid: 0.4, -0.5, -0.6

Figure 10

Inflation-Adjusted Cost of Health Insurance Coverage

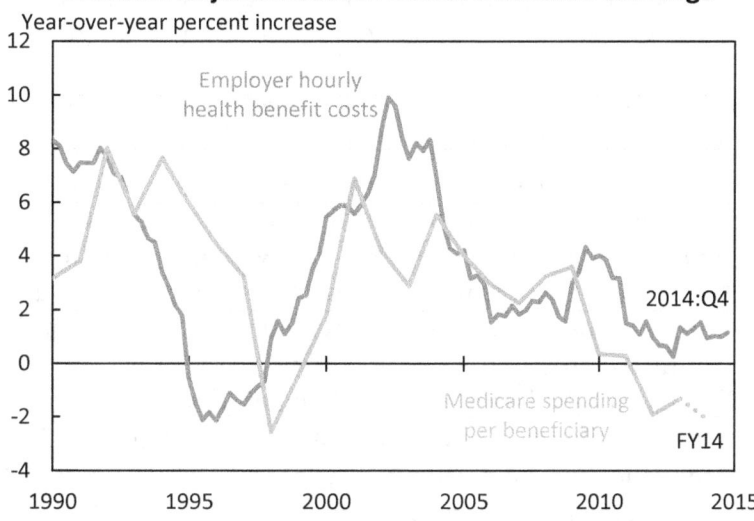

Year-over-year percent increase

Employer hourly health benefit costs

2014:Q4

Medicare spending per beneficiary

FY14

Finally, national health expenditures depend both on the spending per health insurance enrollee as well as on the total number of enrollees—in other words, how many people have health insurance. Through 2013, the slow growth in per-enrollee spending I just mentioned led to very slow growth in aggregate national health expenditures. In particular, the years 2011, 2012, and 2013 are estimated to have seen the slowest growth in real per capita national health expenditures growth since recordkeeping began in 1960.

Despite the fact that per-enrollee spending growth appears to have remained slow during 2014, recent data indicate that aggregate health care spending has begun growing more quickly, likely driven by increased utilization of health care by the roughly ten million people who gained coverage during 2014. A one-time increase in total health care spending as millions gain access

13

to care is both expected and perfectly appropriate since the additional care generates major benefits for the newly insured. Plus, as I noted earlier, this one-time increase in spending is likely helping to accelerate our economic recovery. Finally, it is important to keep in mind that faster aggregate spending growth also does not mean that families who had coverage before 2014 are paying more for care. The costs of care for families who already had coverage depend on trends in prices and per-enrollee spending, which are still rising at unusually slow rates.

The Role of the Affordable Care Act in Recent Cost Trends

The reasons for the recent slow growth in health costs are not yet—and may not ever—be fully understood. CEA has written extensively on its interpretation of recent trends, and I encourage those of you who are interested to seek out CEA's earlier writing on the topic.[15] In brief, the deep recession played some role in recent years' slow growth by causing many to lose coverage and placing pressure on families' and businesses' budgets, leading them to cut back on their demand for health care goods and services, at least in private sector. But the recession cannot provide a complete explanation for the very slow growth in health costs we have seen in recent years. As illustrated in Figure 9, we have seen exceptionally slow growth in Medicare spending alongside slow growth in private health insurance spending, despite the fact Medicare's structure and beneficiaries are relatively insulated from the recession. The fact that slow growth in per-enrollee costs appears to have persisted into 2014, four years into the increasingly strong economic recovery, also suggests that the non-recession factors are playing an important role.

The Affordable Care Act is clearly not the only non-recession factor behind recent slow growth. Long-standing structural factors like rising cost-sharing in private coverage are exerting downward pressure on cost growth, and more transitory factors like sequestration and patent expirations for a number of blockbuster drugs have also contributed to these trends. But it is just as clear that the Affordable Care Act is contributing. One way in which the Affordable Care Act has reduced cost growth in recent years is by reducing excessive payment rates in Medicare. Based on the official score of these provisions by CBO, CEA estimates that the direct effects of these provisions have subtracted around 0.2 percentage points per year from the growth of national health expenditures over the last few years.[16] In addition, Medicare's payment rates often serve as the basis for negotiations between private insurers and providers, and economic research finds that past reductions in Medicare payment rates have generated "spillover" reductions in payment rates in the private sector, suggesting that Affordable Care Act payment changes may have reduced health care spending growth system-wide by around 0.5 percentage

---

[15] (CEA) Council of Economic Advisers. 2014. "Historically Slow Growth in Health Spending Continued in 2013, and Data Show Underlying Slow Cost Growth Is Continuing". December (https://www.whitehouse.gov/blog/2014/12/03/historically-slow-growth-health-spending-continued-2013-and-data-show-underlying-slo); CEA. 2014. *The Economic Report of the President*. March.

[16] CBO estimated that these provisions would reduce Federal outlays by $26 billion in fiscal year 2014, which is around 0.8 percent of national health expenditures in 2014, suggesting an average reduction in NHE growth from these provisions of 0.2 percent per year. Shifting the CBO estimate to a calendar year basis and accounting for the fact that the CBO estimate nets out reductions in beneficiary premium payments and does not include changes in beneficiary cost-sharing would lead to a slightly larger estimate.

points per year.[17] Taken together, these provisions will continue to reduce spending growth by similar amounts in the years ahead.

The Affordable Care Act is also, however, affecting health care delivery in more fundamental ways. As I will discuss in greater detail later, the Affordable Care Act took a variety of steps to begin shifting public sector payment systems away from fee-for-service payment and toward payment models—such as Accountable Care Organizations (ACOs) and bundled payments—that encourage efficient, high-quality care. Prior to the Affordable Care Act, such models were virtually non-existent in Medicare, but, by 2014, about 20 percent of traditional Medicare payments flowed through alternative payment models, all of them created or made possible by the law.

The direct savings in Medicare from these changes have likely been modest so far, but they could be generating larger savings in the private sector. Medicare's position as the largest payer in the Nation's health care system means that when Medicare changes how it pays providers, private payers often follow suit, a point I will return to later. This raises the possibility that by clearly signaling where Medicare will go over the long-term, the Affordable Care Act may already be catalyzing broader changes in the private sector. Indeed, there is evidence that the private sector has made substantial progress on this path in recent years. Private estimates suggest that private payers made around 40 percent of payments through mechanisms other than traditional fee-for-service in 2014, up from an estimated 11 percent in 2013, and have begun entering into ACO-like contracts with providers on a substantial scale.[18]

Recent Improvements in Health Care Quality

Before turning to a more detailed discussion of the economic implications of these encouraging cost trends, I want to remark briefly on recent data on health care quality. While trends in health care costs receive the most attention, trends in health care quality are equally important in determining how the overall economic contribution of the health care sector is changing over time. In fact, if the cost savings were coming at the expense of quality, we would have a different perspective on them, whereas if we were saving money by reducing errors and improving the quality of care, that would be an especially welcome development.

Data on health care quality are scarcer than data on health care costs. And unlike health care spending, where everything is measured in dollars, it is nearly impossible to fully aggregate changes in quality across a variety of different domains. Nevertheless, the data we do have on trends in quality are quite encouraging.

---

[17] Clemens, Jeffrey, and Joshua Gottlieb. 2013. "In the Shadow of a Giant: Medicare's Influence on Private Physician Payments." NBER Working Paper 19503. October; Clemens, Jeffrey, Joshua Gottlieb, and Adam Hale Shapiro. 2014. "How Much Do Medicare Payment Cuts Reduce Inflation?" *Federal Reserve Bank of San Francisco Economic Letter*, vol. 28. September; White, Chapin. 2013. "Contrary to Cost-Shift Theory, Lower Medicare Hospital Payment Rates for Inpatient Care Lead to Lower Private Payment Rates." *Health Affairs* vol. 32, no. 5, pp. 935-943. May.

[18] Catalyst for Payment Reform. 2014. National Scorecard on Payment Reform (http://www.catalyzepaymentreform.org/images/documents/nationalscorecard2014.pdf); Petersen, Matthew, Paul Gardner, Tianna Tu, and David Muhlestein. 2014. Growth and Dispersion of Accountable Care Organizations: June 2014 Update. Leavitt Partners. June.

One of the most comprehensive and systematic ongoing efforts to track health care quality system-wide is the Agency for Healthcare Research and Quality's (AHRQ) work to track the incidence of hospital-acquired conditions, like infections or complications due to medication errors. As depicted in Figure 11, the hospital-acquired condition rate nationwide has fallen 17 percent since AHRQ began tracking these data in 2010. AHRQ estimates that this decline in the rate of patient harm corresponds to 50,000 avoided deaths from 2010 through 2013.

Figure 11

Change in Rate of Patient Harm in U.S. Hospitals

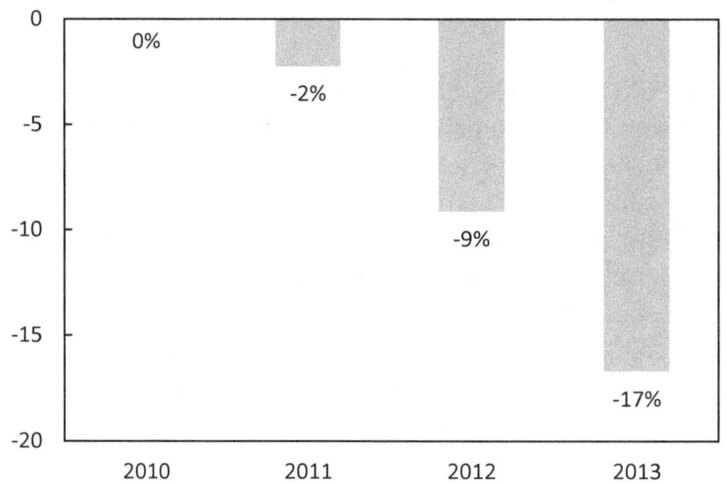

The factors driving the reduction in hospital-acquired conditions are less well-understood than those driving recent trends in costs, but here too aspects of the Affordable Care Act are likely playing a role. Notably, the Affordable Care Act linked hospital's Medicare payment rates to measures of the quality of care they provide through both the Hospital Value-Based Purchasing Program and the Hospital-Acquired Condition Reduction Program. The first year of incentive payments under these programs were based on performance during 2011 and 2013, respectively, and hospitals may also have begun adjusting their behavior even earlier. In addition, the Affordable Care Act created the Partnership for Patients through the Center for Medicare and Medicaid Services, an initiative that helps hospitals identify and diffuse best practices for improving the quality of care. Hospital industry participants have suggested that this program was highly effective in achieving its goals.[19]

The last several years have also seen a sharp reduction in the rate of hospital readmissions, instances in which a patient returns to the hospital soon after discharge. Readmissions are often the result of low-quality care during an initial admission or poor planning for how a patient will receive care after discharge. After having remained approximately flat for several years, 30-day readmission rates fell sharply starting in 2012, a decline that translated into 150,000 avoided readmissions over the period from January 2012 to December 2013.

---

[19] The American Hospital Association/Health Research & Educational Trust Hospital Engagement Network. 2014. *Partnership for Patients Hospital Engagement Network: Final Report*. December.

Figure 12

Medicare 30-Day, All -Condition Hospital Readmission Rate

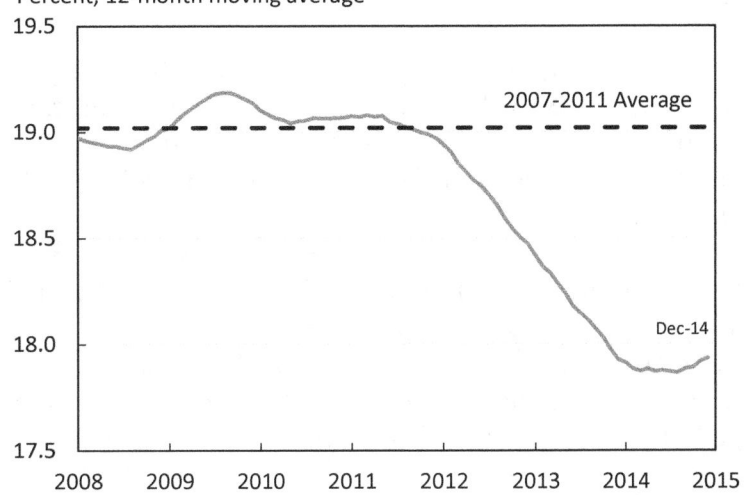
Percent, 12-month moving average

It appears likely that the Affordable Care Act is playing an important role in the recent reduction in readmissions. The Affordable Care Act's Hospital Readmissions Reduction Program reduces payment rates for hospitals in which a relatively large fraction of patients return to the hospital soon after discharge, and the timing of the reduction in readmission rates coincides with the period when this program began to affect hospitals' incentives.[20] The Partnership for Patients may also have contributed to the decline in readmissions during this period by helping hospitals identify and spread strategies for reducing readmissions.

The Benefits of Slower Health Care Cost Growth for the Economy and Our Fiscal Future

As I noted above, the health care sector is more than 17 percent of our overall economy, and every dollar that is spent on health care is a dollar that cannot be used to meet other needs. This means that slower health care cost growth—if achieved without compromising the access to and quality of care, as has been the case over the last few years—generates large improvements in Americans' overall standard of living. These economic benefits show up in two main places: higher wages for people who get coverage through work and lower Federal and State costs.

Benefits for the Labor Market and for Workers

A sizeable majority of non-elderly Americans get health insurance coverage through an employer, which means that much of the benefits of slower health care cost growth will show up as lower premiums in employer-based coverage. Economic theory and evidence demonstrate that, at least in the long run, workers bear the full cost of the coverage they receive, either

---

[20] Many of the rules governing these penalties were finalized in August 2011. The penalties took effect at the start of FY 2013 (October 2012), but because penalties for a given fiscal year are based on hospitals' readmission rates in prior years, hospitals' incentives to begin reducing readmissions began as soon as the rules were finalized (or earlier, to the extent that hospitals anticipated the structure of the payment rules).

directly through premium contributions or indirectly through forgone wages.[21] As a result, slower growth in health insurance premiums in employer-based coverage ultimately translates into larger paychecks for workers.

The amounts of money at stake are quite large. From 2010 through 2014, growth in premiums for employer-based family coverage has been well below 2000-10 average, as measured by the Kaiser Family Foundation and Health Research and Education Trust's Employer Health Benefits Survey. As a result, in 2014, the average family premium was about $1,800 lower than if growth since 2010 had matched the 2000-2010 average.

If slow growth persists in the years ahead, families will realize substantial additional savings. In 2014, growth in the average premium for employer-based family coverage matched the slowest rate since the Kaiser survey began in 1999. If we were able to sustain *just one-third* of the difference between the 2014 growth rate and the 2000-2010 average, then the average family premium would be an additional $2,100 (in 2014 dollars) below the pre-ACA trend by 2020, for a total of nearly $4,000 in savings.

Figure 13

Average Premiums for Employer -Based Family Coverage

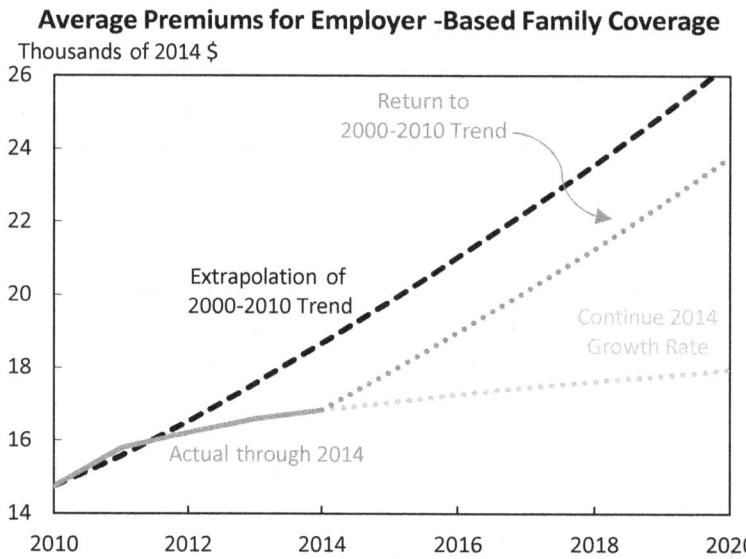

I imagine that almost everyone here agrees that increases in workers' paychecks of this magnitude would be incredibly important. But some, including some of my friends here at CAP, have argued that the savings from slower premium growth are not being passed on to families and are instead accruing to employers.[22] I think this view is mistaken, but it is an important and valid question that deserves a careful answer and continued monitoring in the future.

---

[21] Baicker, Katherine, and Amitabh Chandra. 2006. "The Labor Market Effects of Rising Health Insurance Premiums." *Journal of Labor Economics* vol. 24, no. 3, pp. 609-634; Summers, Lawrence. 1989. "Some Simple Economics of Mandated Benefits." *American Economic Review*, vol. 79, pp. 177–183. May.

[22] Kliff, Sarah. 2015. "Your Company's Health Insurance Costs Are Going Down. But Yours Are Going Up." *Vox*. March (http://www.vox.com/2015/3/11/8190217/health-costs-rising-work); Schoen, Cathy, David Radley, and Sara Collins. 2015. "State Trends in the Cost of Employer Health Insurance Coverage." *The Commonwealth Fund*.

I have seen three main arguments made in favor of this point of view. First, some have argued that the savings families receive from slower premium growth have been consumed by faster growth in their out-of-pocket costs, leaving them no better off. As shown in Figure 14, average deductibles in employer coverage have indeed been growing steadily in recent years. Available data on other types of cost-sharing, like co-payments, suggest that they have increased as well, though not nearly as quickly as deductibles. However, Figure 14 also makes clear that the trend toward higher deductibles stretches back more than a decade, and there is no evidence that this trend has quickened in recent years. That means there is no sense in which continued growth in deductibles is "cancelling out" the slow premium growth of recent years. We are essentially getting the same deductible increases we got before the Affordable Care Act, but much slower premium growth, which is far preferable to the combination that preceded the law.

Figure 14

Average Deductible in Job-Based Single Coverage

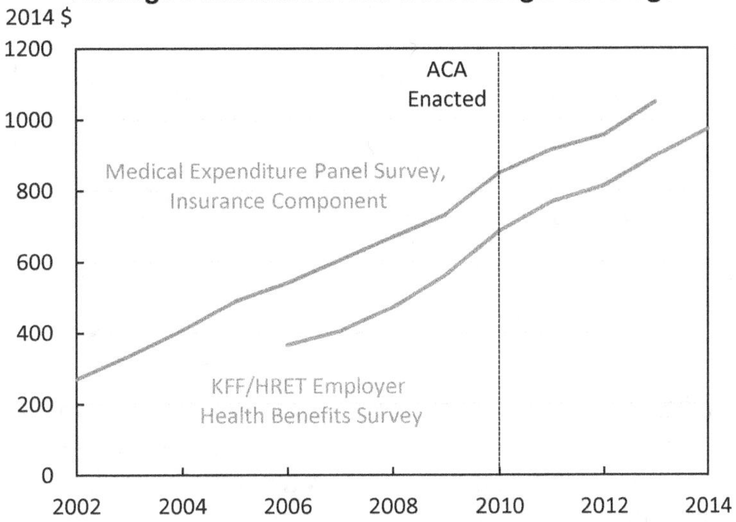

Now, to be clear, I am not arguing that cost-sharing in employer coverage could continue rising indefinitely without raising concerns. While moderate cost-sharing can be an important tool for encouraging people to make efficient use of health care services, excessive cost-sharing can undermine the financial protection that insurance is supposed to provide or keep families from seeking needed care. In fact, the Affordable Care Act abolished lifetime and annual limits on coverage and now requires that all plans place a hard limit on consumers' out-of-pocket spending in order to ensure that everyone with insurance has true protection against catastrophic costs. My point today is that the recent "good news" on premium growth is not a reflection of "bad news" on growth in out-of-pocket costs.

Second, some have suggested that even though overall premium growth has slowed, workers' contributions to premiums have continued to grow rapidly. But this does not appear to be the case. As depicted in Figure 15, workers' premium contributions have, if anything, slowed more

January; Spiro, Topher, Maura Calsyn, and Meghan O'Toole. 2015. "The Great Cost Shift: Why Middle-Class Workers Do Not Feel the Health Care Spending Slowdown." *Center for American Progress*. March.

sharply than total premiums and employers' premium contributions.[23] Indeed, the average worker contribution to family coverage in 2014 was about $900 below what it would have been had growth matched the 2000-2010 trend, indicating that workers have directly captured about half of the $1,800 total savings from slower premium growth over this period, despite the fact that workers directly contribute only a bit more than one-quarter of total premium costs.

Figure 15

Growth in Family Premiums for Job-Based Coverage

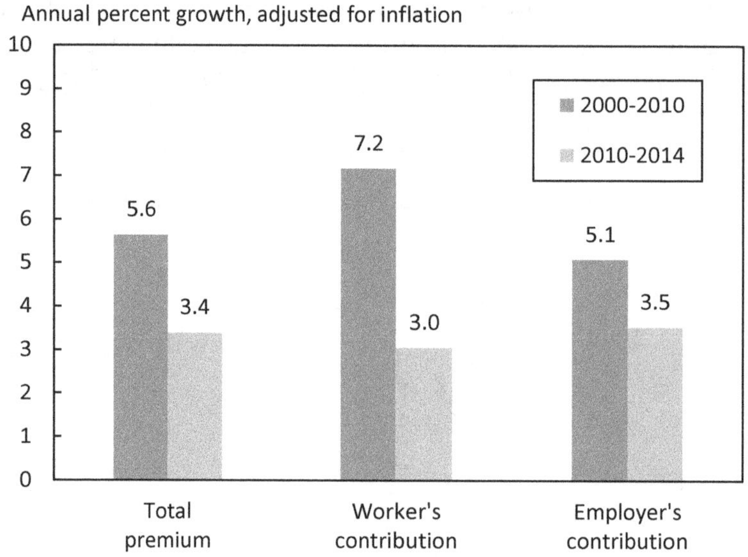

Annual percent growth, adjusted for inflation

Third, some have argued that we are not seeing increases in wage growth commensurate with the slower growth in employers' premium costs. We are, however, seeing a pickup in inflation-adjusted wage growth—with inflation-adjusted wages up at a faster rate in 2013 and 2014 than in the previous economic expansion, as shown in Figure 16. And while the share of economy-wide income that accrues to workers has declined steadily since 2001, it has actually held up better in recent years than it did in the last decade, the opposite of what one would expect if businesses were simply pocketing the premium savings.[24] More fundamentally, we do not know what wage growth would have looked like over the last several years if premium growth had been faster.

---

[23] We use data from the KFF/HRET Employer Health Benefits Survey because data are available through 2014. The Insurance Component of the Medical Expenditure Panel Survey (MEPS-IC), from which data are available through 2013, tells a broadly similar story. In particular, they show that growth in workers' contributions to premiums has slowed to a similar or greater extent than growth in employers' premium contributions. On the other hand, in contrast to the KFF/HRET data, the MEPS-IC data do suggest that growth in workers' premium contributions have grown slightly faster, rather than slightly slower than overall premiums since 2010.

[24] Specifically, the labor share of non-farm business income declined at a rate of 0.1 percent per year from 2010 through 2014, relative to a decline of 0.6 percent per year from 2000 through 2010. Measuring relative to the business cycle trough to control for cyclicality, recent experience still looks slightly better and certainly no worse: the labor share has fallen at a rate of 0.4 percent per year over the 22 quarters following the 2009:Q2 trough, versus 0.5 percent per year over the 22 quarters following the 2001:Q3 trough.

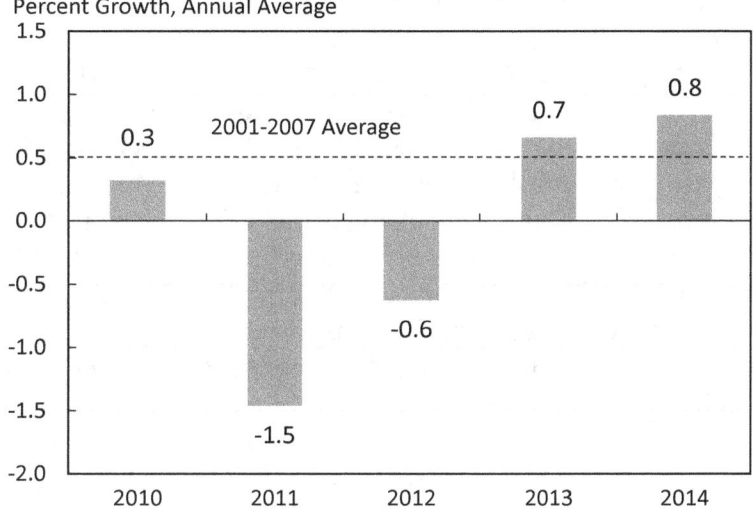

Figure 16
Real Hourly Earnings,
Production & Nonsupervisory Workers

Percent Growth, Annual Average

That said, I am partially sympathetic to this critique. In particular, while economic theory and evidence are clear that employers' premium savings accrue to workers as higher wages in the long run, they do not offer clear guidance on how quickly that will occur. Compensation packages take time to adjust and labor markets take time to reach equilibrium, so it would not be surprising if savings were passed through to wages only gradually. It is also plausible that the pass through to wages has been particularly slow in recent years in the face of the weak labor market we saw in the years immediately following the Great Recession.

If this story is correct, then it has a pair of implications. First, if the money employers have saved on premiums in recent years has not yet been fully passed through to wages, then the scope for wage growth in the years ahead may be larger than it appears, in which case keeping our labor market recovery on track is even more important than it already seemed. Second, it suggests a distinct channel through which slower premium growth may be benefiting workers; namely, if employers have retained a portion of the premium savings, then their per-worker compensation costs are lower than they would otherwise be and their incentives to hire correspondingly higher—precisely the argument made by many advocates of health reform who claimed that the rapid growth of health costs was hurting American job creation. This would imply that slow premium growth is currently boosting employment, helping to accelerate its recovery from the Great Recession. And even in this case, workers would still have gotten the $900 in direct premium savings on their portion of premiums plus higher wages, reflecting at least some portion of the $900 saved by employers.

Benefits for the Nation's Fiscal Future

Federal and State governments are also major beneficiaries of slower growth in health care costs since most Americans who do not get coverage through an employer are covered by either Medicare or Medicaid. Savings to Federal and State governments will generate important economic benefits of their own. For example, if they are used to reduce deficits, they will increase national saving, boosting capital accumulation and reducing foreign borrowing, which raises national income and workers' wages over time. Alternatively, they could be used to finance investments in areas like education or infrastructure, increasing the Nation's productive capacity over the long run, or to cut taxes, increasing families' disposable incomes.

As in the private sector, the potential savings from sustained slow growth in health costs are exceptionally large. Recent changes in CBO projections provide one tangible way of getting a sense of the potential fiscal consequences. In recent years, CBO has concluded that a substantial portion of the slow growth in per-enrollee costs across Medicare, Medicaid, and the private health insurance premiums reflects structural changes that are likely to persist. Largely as a result, CBO has made a series of downward revisions to their projections of Federal spending on major health care programs (Medicare, Medicaid, CHIP, and the Marketplace subsidies). The revisions made from CBO's August 2010 projections through its March 2015 projections have totaled about $1 trillion from 2011-20 and equal $200 billion in 2020—which is about 0.9 percent of projected 2020 GDP.[25]

Figure 17

CBO Projections of Spending on Major Health Care Programs

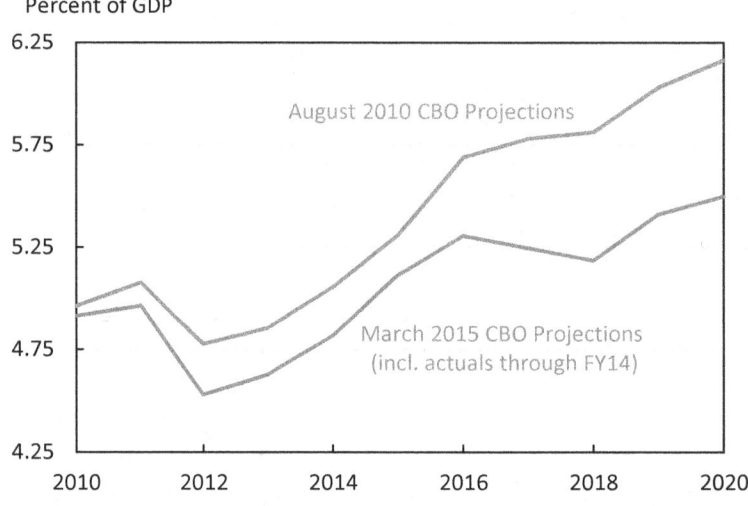

It is important to note that these savings are measured relative to the August 2010 CBO baseline, which already incorporated deficit savings from the Affordable Care Act. CBO's most recent estimate of the overall budgetary effects of the Affordable Care Act is that the law would reduce the deficit by around $100 billion over the period from 2013 to 2022. CBO also estimated that the deficit reduction due to the law would grow rapidly over time, averaging about 0.5 percent of GDP over the subsequent decade (or about $1.6 trillion over that ten-year period).

To put these amounts in context, the Office of Management and Budget estimated earlier this year that the 25-year fiscal gap under current policies—the fiscal adjustment required to stabilize

---

[25] This estimate does not incorporate the House-passed SGR legislation, which will increase Federal health care spending by a bit less than $10 billion in 2020. On the other hand, the $200 billion figure excludes other effects on the Federal budget from reductions in projected health care cost growth, notably reductions in the projected revenue losses to the income and payroll tax exclusion for employer health benefits.

the debt over the next 25 years—was 1.1 percent of GDP.[26] This implies that without the Affordable Care Act and the recent revisions in the long-term outlook for health costs, the Nation's medium-term fiscal problem would be more than twice as large.

Looking Ahead: The Administration's Agenda for Delivery System Reform

It is abundantly clear that our health care system has made major progress over the last several years in expanding coverage, reducing costs, and improving quality, and that progress is having major benefits for our economy. But much remains to be done in all of these areas. I want to focus in the time I have left on the next steps in reforming our health care delivery system, particularly the Administration's strategy for widely deploying new approaches to paying medical providers.

Notably, despite major progress facilitated by the Affordable Care Act, our health care system remains dominated by "fee-for-service" payment systems that pay doctors and hospitals based on the quantity of care they provide, not the outcomes they achieve for patients. Recent evidence has bolstered the case that alternative ways of paying medical providers can generate substantial improvements in the efficiency and quality of patient care. Facilitating the wide deployment of these models is likely the best tool we have to ensure that recent progress on costs and quality— and the economic benefits that come with that progress—continues in the years ahead.

The Case for Adopting Alternative Payment Models

The deficiencies of fee-for-service payment are likely familiar to many of those in the audience today, but, in brief, economists agree that traditional fee-for-service payment systems have at least three troubling consequences for the care patients receive.[27] First, fee-for-service payment leads to excessive use of low-value services since health care providers' incomes are tied directly to the number of services they provide. Second, it provides little or no direct financial incentive to improve quality of care since payments do not vary based the quality of the care patients receive. Third, fee-for-service payment encourages poorly-coordinated care since each provider a patient sees is paid separately and no single provider has a financial incentive to make sure that the overall package of care a patient receives fits together as a coherent whole.

These shortcomings of fee-for-service are why the Administration is using the tools created by the Affordable Care Act to widely deploy "alternative payment models" that orient payment around an episode of care or the patient as a whole, rather than individual services. In doing so, these payment models support care coordination and eliminate the incentive to provide excessive services. These models also generally link payment to quality performance in order to encourage the provision of high-quality care.

---

[26] Office of Management and Budget. 2016. *Analytical Perspectives, Budget of the United States Government, Fiscal Year 2016.*

[27] For a more detailed discussion, see Furman, Jason, and Matt Fiedler. 2015. "Continuing the Affordable Care Act's Progress on Delivery System Reform Is an Economic Imperative." March (https://www.whitehouse.gov/blog/2015/03/24/continuing-affordable-care-act-s-progress-delivery-system-reform-economic-imperative).

Alternative payment models can take a variety of forms, but two prominent examples include bundled payments and "accountable care" payment models. Bundled payments are currently undergoing a large-scale test through the Center for Medicare and Medicaid Innovation, which was created by the Affordable Care Act. Under this model, Medicare makes a single payment for all services associated with an episode of care, like a hip replacement. In the most comprehensive version of bundled payment being tested by the Innovation Center, the bundle includes physician and hospital services during the initial hospital stay, as well as services delivered during a period after the hospital stay.[28] More than 6,000 hospitals, physician groups, and post-acute care providers are engaged in this project and initial results will become available over the coming year.

The Affordable Care Act has also widely deployed "accountable care" models in which providers take on the responsibility for managing the cost and quality of all of a patient's care during the year and can earn "shared savings" if they reduce average per-person spending below a benchmark level while also delivering high-quality care. Across the country, medical providers have formed 424 ACOs serving 7.8 million Medicare beneficiaries through the Innovation Center's Pioneer ACO Program and the Medicare Shared Savings Program, both made possible by the Affordable Care Act.

Experience with alternative payment models is still relatively limited, but evidence to date is promising. Perhaps the best evidence on the potential of such models comes from research on from Blue Cross Blue Shield of Massachusetts' Alternative Quality Contract (AQC), which has been operating since 2009 and is similar to the two-sided risk ACO contracts offered by Medicare.[29] This study found that the AQC found that gross per-patient claims costs of AQC-participating providers fell markedly relative to similar providers in comparison States, generating gross savings of 10 percent by the fourth year that the contract was in use. AQC-participating providers also markedly improved quality relative to the comparison group.

While the gross savings were outweighed by bonus payments to providers in the early years of the AQC, the AQC generated net savings by its fourth year. Furthermore, the structure of the AQC in its early years may have led to higher bonus payments than were actually necessary to ensure participation in the contract, suggesting that other approaches to accountable care could generate larger net savings. Regardless, the AQC experience provides strong evidence that accountable care models can generate large positive changes in medical practice.

---

[28] In practice, under this model, Medicare pays each of the providers involved in the patient's care separately via the existing fee-for-service system, then reconciles those amounts against the bundled payment after the fact. The economic incentives created by this approach are virtually identical to those under a "prospective" bundled payment.
[29] Song, Zirui, Sherri Rose, Dana Safran, Bruce Landon, Matthew Day, and Michael Chernew. 2014. "Changes in Health Care Spending and Quality 4 Years into Global Payment." *The New England Journal of Medicine*, vol. 371, pp. 1704-1714. October.

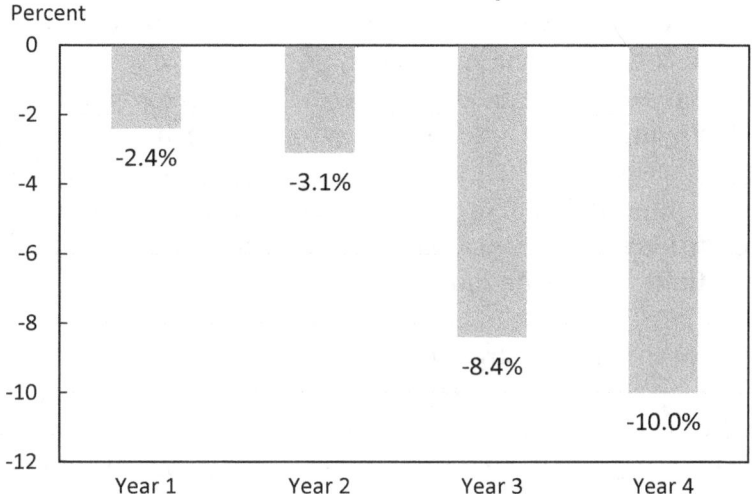

Figure 18
Change in Gross Per-Patient Claims Costs
Under the Alternative Quality Contract

The Administration's Strategy for Widely Deploying Alternative Payment Models

Widely deploying alternative payment models is likely the best tool we have to ensure that recent progress toward reducing costs and improving quality continues. The Administration has a three-pronged strategy to achieve that outcome.

First, HHS plans to move aggressively to deploy these models in Medicare. As I noted earlier, about 20 percent of traditional Medicare payments flowed through alternative payment models in 2014, up from virtually none before the law passed. HHS has set the goal of making further progress in the years ahead, with 30 percent of traditional Medicare payments flowing through these models by 2016 and 50 percent by 2018.

Deploying these models in Medicare is important in its own right, but historical experience and economic evidence implies that doing so will also help accelerate their deployment system-wide. Medicare is the Nation's single largest payer, so it has a unique ability to engage providers to deploy new models, which other payers can then capitalize on. For example, when Medicare deployed "prospective payment" for hospitals during the 1980s, private payers followed suit. More recently, economic research has found that when Medicare changed the structure of how it paid physicians, private payment patterns followed suit.[30]

Nevertheless, action by public programs may not be sufficient to ensure widespread adoption of new payment models in the private sector. Economic research in a variety of settings has found that when one payer changes its practices in ways that reduce costs or improve quality, other payers in the same market may benefit as well since medical providers apply the improved

---

[30] Clemens, Jeffrey, and Joshua Gottlieb. 2013. "In the Shadow of a Giant: Medicare's Influence on Private Physician Payments." NBER Working Paper No. 19503. October.

approaches to care delivery with all of their patients.[31] For example, research on the AQC has found that Medicare realized "spillover" cost savings as the AQC came online for privately-insured patients in Massachusetts.[32]

The presence of cross-payer "spillovers" means that the deployment of alternative payment models can face a classic collective action problem, in which all payers are better off in a world where alternative payment models are the norm, but many payers would rather let someone else do the hard work of deploying them. Collaborative effort between public and private payers may be able to help solve this problem by helping payers agree to move forward together or by facilitating the spread of information in order reduce adoption costs. Collaborative efforts may also make it easier for different payers to align their new models, reducing administrative costs for providers and potentially increasing models' efficacy.

Thus, the second prong of the Administration's strategy is to find ways to facilitate this type of collaborative work across payers. Toward that end, HHS has created a Health Care Payment Learning and Action Network that brings together public- and private-sector stakeholders to work to address these barriers. The Network met at the White House for the first time last week and meetings will continue in the months ahead.

Third, the President's Fiscal Year 2016 budget included the bicameral, bipartisan proposal from 2014 to reform Medicare's broken Sustainable Growth Rate (SGR) physician payment system. In addition to permanently eliminating the risk of steep cuts in Medicare physician payment rates, this bill, which recently passed in the House and will soon come up in the Senate, would more strongly link Medicare's fee-for-service physician payment rates to providers' efficiency and quality, while also providing incentives that encourage physicians to participate in alternative payment models. Both of these steps will catalyze the Administration's other delivery system reform efforts, and, as the President has said, he looks forward to signing a good bipartisan bill.

I will also note that, in addition to fixing Medicare's physician payment system and advancing delivery system reform, this legislation will make progress in several other high-priority areas. Notably, the legislation will continue CHIP, protect access to care through Community Health Centers, and extend the proven Maternal, Infant, and Early Childhood Home Visiting Programs. At the same time, the legislation enacts sensible reforms similar to proposals in the President's Budget that will offset costs above what is needed to hold Medicare payments to physicians fixed at their current level and a larger share of the legislation's long-run costs. These include cost-saving changes to Medicare provider payments, increases in income-related premiums for certain high-income Medicare beneficiaries that reduce the Federal subsidy of Medicare costs for

[31] Baicker, Katherine, Michael Chernew, and Jacob Robbins. 2013. "The Spillover Effects of Medicare Managed Care: Medicare Advantage and Hospital Utilization." *Journal of Health Economics* vol. 32, no. 6, pp. 1289-1300. December; Glied, Sherry, and Joshua Graff Zivin. 2002. "How do Doctors Behave When Some (But Not All) of Their Patients Are in Managed Care?" *Journal of Health Economics*, vol. 21, no. 2, pp. 337-353. March.
[32] McWilliams, Michael, Bruce Landon, and Michael Chernew. 2013. "Changes in Health Care Spending and Quality for Medicare Beneficiaries Associated with a Commercial ACO Contract." *Journal of the American Medical Association* vol. 310, no. 8, pp. 829-836. August.

those who need the subsidy the least, and limits on coverage of the Part B deductible in Medigap plans for future beneficiaries that will encourage more efficient use of health care.

Conclusion

Looking back over five years of the Affordable Care Act, the evidence is clear: not only have the doomsday predictions of the law's critics been decisively refuted by events, but the Affordable Care Act is working to expand coverage, reduce costs, and improve quality—all of which are also helping our economy. But the law's work is not done, nor is the work that remains self-executing. In the years ahead, the Administration will use the law's tools and the knowledge we are gaining from it operation to make further progress, particularly by continuing our efforts to move toward a health care delivery system that consistently provides efficient, high-quality care.

Notes to Figures and Tables

Figure 1
Source: Bureau of Labor Statistics; CEA calculations.

Figure 2
Source: Bureau of Labor Statistics; CEA calculations.

Figure 3
Source: Congressional Budget Office; CEA calculations
Note: 2019 is the last year covered in the March 2010 estimates. The GDP estimates underlying CBO's March 2010 estimates have been adjusted for major NIPA revisions in the summer of 2013. Without these revisions, the decline since March 2010 would be larger.

Figure 4
Source: CEA analysis of National Health Interview Survey, Cohen et al. (2009), Klemm (2000), and CMS (2009); ASPE analysis of NHIS and Gallup-Healthways Well-Being Index data through March 4, 2015.
Note: Data are quarterly starting in 2014:Q1. Data for earlier years are generally either annual or bi-annual. The NHIS is the best tool for studying trends in insurance coverage, but because NHIS data are not currently available after 2014:Q3, Gallup data are used to extrapolate the uninsured rate through 2015:Q1.

Figure 5
Source: Current Population Survey, Annual Social and Economic Supplement, 2014.

Figure 6
Source: National Health Interview Survey; CEA calculations.

Figure 7
Source: Bureau of Labor Statistics; Gallup-Healthways Well-Being Index; CEA calculations.

Note: In most states, we include only employment in the health care services industry. For seven states, health care services employment is reported jointly with social assistance employment, and for these states we use the broader category. No data are available for New Mexico.

Figure 8
Source: Bureau of Economic Analysis; CEA calculations.

Figure 9
Source: Centers for Medicare and Medicaid Services; Bureau of Economic Analysis; CEA calculations.

Figure 10
Source: Centers for Medicare and Medicaid Services; Bureau of Labor Statistics; Bureau of Economic Analysis; Congressional Budget Office; CEA calculations.
Note: The 2014 figure is a CBO estimate for fiscal year 2014 that was adjusted for timing shifts by CBO. All other figures are calendar year CMS estimates. The growth rate for 2006 excludes prescription drug expenditures to avoid distortions from the creation of Medicare Part D.
Figure 11
Source: Agency for Health Care Research and Quality; CEA calculations.

Figure 12
Source: Centers for Medicare and Medicaid Services, Office of Enterprise Data and Analytics; CEA calculations.

Figure 13
Source: Kaiser Family Foundation and Health Research and Education Trust, Employer Health Benefits Survey; Bureau of Economic Analysis; CEA calculations.

Figure 14
Source: Kaiser Family Foundation and Health Research and Education Trust, Employer Health Benefits Survey; Agency for Healthcare Research and Quality, Medical Expenditure Panel Survey; Bureau of Economic Analysis; CEA calculations.

Figure 15
Source: Kaiser Family Foundation and Health Research and Education Trust, Employer Health Benefits Survey; Bureau of Economic Analysis; CEA calculations.

Figure 16
Source: Bureau of Labor Statistics, Current Employment Statistics; CEA calculations.

Figure 17
Source: Congressional Budget Office; CEA calculations.
Note: The August 2010 GDP estimates have been adjusted for major NIPA revisions in the summer of 2013. Without these revisions, the decline since August 2010 would be larger.

Figure 18

Source: Song et al., 2014.